Low Carb Diet

Lose Weight and Never Gain it Back with These Easy Low Carb Recipes

Introduction

I'd like to thank you for downloading the book, *"Low Carb Diet"*.

This book teaches you all about a low carb diet and gives you some delicious low carb recipes.

Do you wish to make your weight loss process effortless and quick? Do you want to be super-healthy without eating less? Do you intend to combat diabetes and several other health conditions? If yes, then the perfect solution to all your problems is a 'low carb diet.'

This book provides you with details on what a low-carb diet is, its benefits and also offers you some amazing low-carb recipes for breakfast, lunch, dinner and dessert, to get you started on the diet without any problem. Get started with it now to unlock a healthier, happier life.

Thanks again for downloading this book, I hope you enjoy it!

3

Table of Contents

Understanding A Low-Carb Diet

A low-carb diet is extremely healthy and benefits your body in a number of ways. Discover what it actually is, and why you should opt for this wonderful diet.

What Is A Low Carb Diet?

A low-carb diet is simply a diet that is low in carbs or carbohydrates and emphasizes more on consuming foods rich in fat and protein, which is why it is also sometimes referred to as a high-fat or high-protein diet. When on a low-carb diet, you are required to limit your consumption of foods rich in carbs, such as starchy fruit, starchy veggies, pasta, bread, beans, rice, potatoes and grains.

However, you can eat high-protein and high-fat foods. (The list is given below.) There are a number of low-carb diets, such as ketogenic, Scarsdale, Stillman, Hollywood and Atkins diet. They vary according to the amount of carbs, fat and protein you can consume while on the diet.

How Much Can You Eat When Following This Diet?

There is no restriction on exactly how much you can eat when you are on a low-carb diet. You can eat whenever you feel hungry. There's absolutely no need to keep measuring how many calories you consume, or even weigh your food before you eat it. However, what you need to pay special attention to is the amount of carbohydrates you can eat. If you are active, lean and have a high metabolic rate, and want to use the low-carb diet to maintain your current weight, you can consume about 100g to around 150g of carbs per day, but it is best to stay around 100g. If you intend to make your weight loss process quick and efficient, and restrict your carb intake, it is best to stick to about 50g to 100g of carbs per day. However, if you have diabetes, or are metabolically slow, or want to lose weight super-fast, you should consume about 20g to 50g of carbohydrates daily.

How A Low-Carb Diet Works?

Your body is designed to use energy from glucose when carbohydrates are broken down. Therefore, when you are on a high-carb diet, your body gets its energy from glucose. As glucose levels rise, more insulin is secreted by your pancreas. Insulin stimulates the cells to use the glucose for energy. The excess glucose gets converted into glycogen by the enzyme glucagon which works as your body's energy reserve. When you cut back on your carb intake, your body starts to use those glycogen reserves. Soon, those reserves deplete and can no longer satisfy your body's energy needs. At this point, the mitochondria in your liver uses acetyl CoA to produce ketones which are organic molecules comprising of a carbon atom linked with one oxygen atom via a double bond, and also linked with two carbon units too. Meanwhile, it starts to use the stored fat in your body to satiate its energy demands, which is why your body breaks down fat quickly and you lose weight. As the ketone levels of your body increase, your body enters the state of 'ketosis.' Your brain and body use ketones to get energy. As the ketones level increases, your body becomes dependent on them for energy. Furthermore, since you take in very little carbohydrate, there is little to no extra glucose in your body and your blood sugar level does not spike. Moreover, hardly any glucose gets converted to glycogen and fat, so you don't gain more weight.

Why adopt the low-carb diet? Is the low carb diet for you? Let us address this in the following chapter.

Why Go On A Low-Carb Diet?

Now, that you have a basic understanding of a low-carb diet, it's time to find out why you need to try this diet.

It trains your body to burn more fat: When you restrict your intake of carbohydrates, your blood sugar level starts to stabilize. When sugar levels stabilize, the insulin levels drop too. As a result, less glucose is stored in the muscles and fat cells in your body. When there are fewer glycogen reserves to use, your body begins to burn more fat reserves to get energy, which results in the burning of more calories and hence enhances weight loss. **Numerous studies** back up this fact.

Makes you feel satiated quickly: When you reduce your consumption of carbohydrates, your blood sugar level stabilizes which means you experience less sugar spikes (known to increase your level of craving to eat) than before. Moreover, as your body becomes carbohydrate deficient, the mitochondria in your liver produce ketones to fulfill your energy needs. The increased production of ketones usually results in a **rise in the level of CCK (cholecystokinin), a hormone responsible for making you feel satiated** and satisfied. Therefore, when you consume more fat and protein, you become full easily and quickly without eating a lot. Moreover, **ketones also promote the reduction of ghrelin in your body,** which is a hormone that boosts your hunger.

You become more energetic and efficient: When you consume more carbs, you supply your body with a constant stream of energy. When your body knows it has endless reserves of glycogen, it becomes lazy and inefficient. On the other hand, when you consume less carbs and more fat, your body becomes forced to mobilize fats to get energy. This sudden change encourages it to work harder and efficiently, which improves your energy levels and makes you energetic.

Decreases Insulin Resistance: When your body gets too much glucose, its **insulin level rises**. When the insulin levels in your body skyrocket, your cells soon becomes resistant to insulin; thus, this forces your body to produce more insulin to deal with the high carbohydrate intake and, over time, you become insulin resistant, which is a precursor for type II diabetes. However, if you **shift to a low-carb diet, you manage the insulin levels in your body** and gradually decrease your body's resistance to insulin, which helps you manage your diabetes and become healthy.

Weight Loss: In 2014, the National institute of health carried out a study that tried to figure out which diet is good for weight loss. In this study, they observed 148 people who were taking low-carb foods and high-fat foods over a period of 12 months. They then discovered that a low-carb diet was more effective and superior when it came to weight loss and the reduction of cardiovascular risk factor.

The reason why low-carb diets are very effective when it comes to weight loss is because they help your body to get rid of the number one enemy of weight loss, which is insulin also known as the fat–storage hormone. As you read earlier, insulin usually signals all the cells to store as much fat as they can for later use, and so, with low levels of insulin, your body turns to fat as its main source of energy. When this happens, your body becomes a fat burning machine that burns every possible fat in your body. This leads to great weight loss.

What To Eat And What To Avoid?

Here is a list of all the foods you can to eat when on this diet.

Foods You Can Eat

Fish: You can eat all sorts of fatty fish, including mackerel, herring, and salmon.

Meat: You can eat chicken, pork, beef, game meat as well as the chicken skin and fat. It is best to go for grass-fed or organic meat.

Eggs: You can eat organic eggs cooked in various ways.

Vegetables: You can eat cabbage, Brussels sprouts, eggplant, zucchini, spinach, peppers, onions, mushrooms, tomatoes, cucumber, asparagus and all the veggies that grow above the ground.

Fat Sources: You can consume natural fat sources, such as organic butter and cream, olive oil and coconut oil.

Dairy Foods: You can consume full-fat options such as sour cream, real butter, Turkish/ Greek yogurt and all sorts of high-fat cheeses. Try to limit your intake of skim and regular milk, as they are high in milk sugar.

Berries: You can have them (blackberries, strawberries, blueberries, raspberries etc.) in moderation, but make sure not to consume them daily.

Nuts: Cashew nuts, pistachio, almonds, walnuts, sunflower seeds, Macadamia Nuts, and other nuts high in fat content.

In addition to berries, you can eat other fruits low in sugar like avocados, apples and any other fruit that does not have too much sugar like watermelon, cantaloupe, peaches, star fruit, kiwi, cherries, plum and honeydew. The thing about fruits is that they contain fructose, a form of sugar, which can easily spike your blood sugar levels and make it hard for you to lose weight effectively, as the body prefers simple sugars (fructose is a simple sugar) to other energy sources.

In addition to these foods, you can drink tea and coffee. Make sure to increase your water intake when on a low-carb diet.

Foods to Avoid

Sugar: All foods and beverages high in sugar, such as sweet chocolate, buns, pastries, juices, energy drinks, breakfast cereals and sweeteners are prohibited on this diet.

Margarine: This is an industrial imitation of butter and is rich in unhealthy fats, which is why you must avoid it while on a low-carb diet.

Starch Foods: Rice, bread, potatoes, pasta, muesli, porridge, legumes, root vegetables, and even wholegrain products should be avoided when you follow a low-carb diet.

Fruit: With a low carb diet, we are looking to lower your intake of carbohydrates. All fruits are rich in sugar (fructose); thus, you need to limit your fruit intake greatly. Just eat a fruit or two in a week and try not to do more than that.

Beer and Alcohol: Avoid all kinds of beer and alcoholic beverages.

Initial Side-Effects And Tips To Overcome Them

Although a low-carb diet is highly beneficial for you, you do tend to experience a few side effects in the first few days since your body is not used to depending on fat for energy. Here are the different side effects you may experience in the beginning along with tips to overcome them easily.

1. Fatigue, headaches, dizziness and irritability

The above are the side effects that you will probably experience in your first week - more specifically between the second and the fourth day. These symptoms are usually caused by dehydration or salt deficiency that comes from a temporary increase in urine production that is usually caused by the cutting back of carbohydrate consumption. The good news is that these symptoms tend to disappear by themselves over time.

2. Constipation

The constipation is usually brought about by dehydration, which sucks water out of your intestines and leaves your stomach with dry and hard food content. Below are ways to deal with the constipation:

Drink plenty of fluids: This will make sure that you have adequate water and even if some water is sucked from the intestines, you still have a little water to ensure you have a smooth digestion process.

Eat more fiber rich foods: High quality fiber intake keeps your intestines moving smoothly and that can help you avoid constipation. Good sources of fiber rich foods include non-starchy vegetables.

3. Leg cramps

The leg cramps are usually caused by a loss of minerals like magnesium that occur due to increased urination. Below is what you can do to deal with the leg cramps:

Drink lots of water and get enough salt*:* By drinking plenty of fluids, your body will get more water than it actually loses. That will automatically reduce the loss of magnesium.

Take some magnesium supplements: You can replace magnesium loss by taking magnesium supplement tablets like Mag 64 or Slow-Mag once a day for 20 days.

4. Increased Heart Rate

Increased heart rate is another common side-effect that occurs during your first few weeks on a low carb diet. This is usually caused by the lack of circulating fluids in your blood stream that forces your heart to pump blood harder than it used to in order to maintain blood pressure. The two things that lead to the reduction of circulating fluids are lack of salt in your body and dehydration. Therefore, drink more water and increase your salt intake.

5. Reduction in physical performance

More often than not, you are likely not to be in your top shape during the first few weeks while on a low carb diet. There are two reasons why this happens. The first reason is the lack of enough fluid, which is likely to lead to dehydration. To avoid this, you should drink a lot of water - probably 1 large glass with a teaspoon of salt every one hour. The second reason why your body might experience reduced physical performance is because your body will take time to adapt from using glucose for energy to burning fat for energy. Thus, give your body some time to adapt to burning fat for energy.

If you are a beginner, it is best to go slow and easy on this diet, and adapt to it over a period of four to five weeks. This gives your body enough time to adjust to the shift, so you experience fewer side effects.

Switching to a Low Carb Diet

You might experience a little difficulty while shifting to the low carb diet, as it will mean not being able to indulge in some of your favorite foods. But remember that most of the challenges can be easily overcome with just a little effort from your end.

To help you transition into the diet, here are some simple tips to follow.

Counting Carbs

You must calculate your carb intake, as it cannot be forgone. Make this a habit right from the start so that it becomes a lasting habit. Start off by introducing small changes such as reading the labels on the packs and ensure that you can adjust the carbs into your diet. Make it a point to go through all the labels regardless of the food item. Take a friend along who can remind you to check the labels before buying the packs. You have to look at the net carbs mentioned on the pack. Net carbs = total carbs - fiber.

Avoid sugar alcohols as much as possible. You are allowed to consume no more than 20 net carbs per day. This can change a little but should not go past 30 per day. If you happen to work out regularly, then 30 net carbs are allowed. Your body will also be able to produce a good dose of ketones that can be drawn up for energy. You can download an app that will help you keep track of the number of calories that you consume.

Clear the kitchen

One of the best ways to get started with the diet is by clearing out the kitchen and getting rid of all temptations. Most people who adopt a diet tend to easily fall prey to unhealthy foods that will be present in their kitchens. If there are chocolates, candies, sodas, bread, etc. then you will feel like eating them and end up breaking the flow of the diet. So, make sure you kick these out of your kitchen and replace them with healthier options.

Eating out

When you first take up the ketogenic diet, you have to make sure you bear in mind the restaurants that you go to. Before you go to the restaurant, have a look at its menu to determine whether there are meals that are low carb friendly. Make sure you know how many calories you are allowed to consume beforehand so that it becomes easier to order at the restaurant. To help you out, here are some meals that you can consider ordering at a restaurant.

Order eggs for breakfast. They are full of proteins and low on carbs. You can order omelets or boiled eggs and bacon. For lunch, go for lean meat recipes such as chicken salad and consume it with a bowl of greens. Give the salad dressing a skip as it can contain sugar. If you do not like salads, then go for a healthy fish dish along with vegetables on the side. For dinner, you can order a lean meat dish. Go for green vegetables and some low carb bread. Avoid sides such as possible especially fries and wedges. If you wish to have potatoes, then go for baked options.

Ready snacks

Most of us are guilty of going for snacks that are high in carbs. We tend to reach out to them during our hunger pangs and end up forgoing calorie counting. To avoid this, you have to pile up on some low carb snacks that you can reach for when you start feeling puckish.

- Vegetable sticks with a Greek yogurt dip. Right from celery sticks to beetroot to carrot sticks, you can cut them into long, slender sticks and consume them with a natural Greek yogurt dip. Season it using salt and pepper to flavor the dip.
- Nuts happen to be great snacking options when you take up the low carb diet. Right from walnuts to cashew nuts to groundnuts, there are many choices. Make sure you

toast them a little so that they can last longer. Avoid readymade nuts as they can contain sugars, salt and oils.

- Healthy chips made using kale. All you have to do is cut the kale into thin slices and add a little oil to a pan. Allow it to heat up before adding in the kale and browning it thoroughly on all sides. You can also consider placing it in an oven dish and drizzling some oil over it before adding to the oven to crisp up.

Ketosis

When you take up a low carb diet, your body undergoes a process known as ketosis. Ketosis is an important process that helps in providing the body with the energy required to carry out day-to-day activities. It replaces the carbs in the diet and makes sure your body does not get too much of it. For this, you can check whether your body has entered a state of ketosis so that you can maintain the diet.

You can buy a ketosis stick that is used to check the level of ketosis occurring in your body. You are required to add a few drops of your urine on the stick to know your level of ketosis. If the color turns dark purple, then it indicates a high level of ketones present in your body. This is not a healthy sign, as you must aim at a color that is light purple and dark pink. That is when you will lose quite a bit of weight. Do not drink too much water before taking the test, as you will end up diluting your urine. At the same time, you should not deny your body of water, as dehydration will not give you an accurate reading.

As you can see, there are many simple things that you can do to stick with a low carb diet. Place a reminder on your phone to calculate your calories before every meal, and you are sure to stick with your diet and make it a success.

Sticking to the Diet

Once you successfully transition into the diet, it becomes essential for you to take measures to stick with it. This is easier said than done, as most people tend to go off a diet after a few months of starting out. If you wish to avoid this from happening then here are some things that you can do to stick with the diet and continue with it for a long time.

Research

Make sure you do your research and prepare yourself for the journey that lies ahead. Go through all the material that is available on the topic and prepare yourself. This book will provide you with a lot of material no doubt but do not limit yourself to just this, go through other resources as well to increase your knowledge on the subject. Go through testimonials of people who have tried the diet and what they have to say about it. Find websites that mention the benefits of the diet and how it can help women lose weight easily. You can join in with a group in your area where people, who have taken up the diet, meet and discuss it.

Recipes

One good way of keeping your interest up is by buying a recipe book. It is apparent that you will not be able to come up with new recipes by yourself and will require a little help. In such a case, you can buy a book and look up recipes that you can try out. There are also many websites that provide good recipes that you can try out and stick with the diet. As and when you get the hang of it, you will begin to prepare ketogenic dishes on your own. You can use the recipes mentioned in this book as inspiration and come up with recipes of your own. All you have to do is mix and match the ingredients.

Stay inspired

One important thing to do is to remain inspired to stick with the diet for life. One way of keeping up with the diet is by speaking to someone who has experienced positive results with the diet. Ask them about their journey and how they managed to use the diet to get the positive benefits. Once you understand it, you can start a campaign of your own and write about your daily experiences and the benefits that you are getting from the diet. Click pictures of yourself and keep posting it so that you can share your journey with others and use it as a means to stay inspired.

Partner up

A partner can help you not only stick with the diet but also make it easier to prepare the dishes and take up exercise routines. Ask your husband, partner or a friend to join in and keep you company during the diet. With time, you will be able to turn it into a lifestyle choice. Your partner can share in the responsibilities and cook meals for both.

Keep track

Remember always to keep track of your journey and measure your progress. Right from the amount of weight that you lose to your vital statistics, you have to keep track of how you are progressing. Get a basic test done through your GP before starting out on the diet and then take one three months into it. You will see that your blood pressure has normalized, your blood glucose is in control, your stamina has increased and so has your energy.

Patience

You have to remain patient and not expect to see overnight results. Give the diet at least a month to work its magic on you. Once the ball gets rolling, and you notice a certain weight loss, you will feel motivated to go on with the diet for life.

These are just some ways in which you can remain motivated with the diet and not limited to just these. You can try out other things as well so that you have the best chance to turn the diet into a lifestyle choice.

How the Low Carb Diet Works

The low-carb diet is a great diet to incorporate to lose weight and maintain a fit body. There is scientific backing to prove that the low carb diet works for pretty much anyone who takes it up.

There have been 23 studies on humans to showcase how effective the diet is. In fact, the results have been extremely pleasing thereby rendering the low carb diet one of the best in the world for weight loss. In most cases, a low-carb diet leads to three times the weight loss, as the low-fat content helps in developing a fitter body. The low carb diet is highly recommended, as it has no significant side effects on people. This makes it a lucrative choice for people to consider. In fact, many studies have shown that the diet helps in reversing several health conditions and can promote wellness among all who take up the diet.

The triglycerides in the body are reduced, and the HDL is raised. A person's blood pressure levels are regularized thereby contributing towards good heart health. Blood sugar levels are also taken care of therefore ensuring that diabetes risk is considerably reduced.

A large percentage of the fat that is lost through the low carb diet is from the stomach region. This fat is better known as visceral fat and can be quite dangerous for the body. This fat is tough to get rid of, and so, only a particular diet like the low carb diet can help people lose this fat. If this fat is not taken out, then it can negatively impact the organs that surround the stomach such as liver and heart and lead to illnesses.

The low carb diet has been shown to help people who suffer from metabolic illnesses and Type 2 diabetes. There has been enough evidence to prove that the diet can efficiently minimize the risk of both these diseases. To help you understand exactly how effective this diet is and what can be done to make the most of its effects, here is a look at the different health benefits that it provides.

Insulin control

The insulin is a hormone secreted in the body by the pancreas. Insulin happens to be one of the essential hormones in the body as it helps in synthesizing blood sugar. When a person consumes a carb-rich or sugar-laden meal, then the blood sugar levels spike up. The insulin is released to bind with the sugar and turn it into energy-providing molecules. But if the person ends up consuming far too much sugar then it leads to insulin dysfunction. Insulin also has the function of informing the fat cells in the body to produce fat and store it. In the event of a malfunction, the cells get confused and start storing more and more fat assuming that the body has entered a state of emergency. The body fails to pick the glucose from the bloodstream and ends up storing it as fat. In such a case, it is best to choose a low carb diet where the number of carbs is limited. This helps in controlling the insulin levels secreted in the body. The insulin stimulates and inhibits lipolysis or the burning of fat in the body. As the carbs are restricted, the insulin levels gradually reduce, and the fat cells get used up to provide energy for the body. So the diet goes a long way in helping people manage their insulin levels and control diabetes.

Water weight

Within the first couple of weeks of taking on the diet, your water weight begins to reduce drastically. Here is a look at the process.

- When the insulin levels go down, the kidney starts to lose excess sodium from the body and ends up lowering the blood pressure.
- Carbs in the body are stored in the form of glycogen. This glycogen binds with water in muscles and liver. When the carb input reduces, the glycogen level goes down and so does the water.

This does not occur on a diet that is high in carbs even if the calories are reduced.

But there will be some who will not consider water weight as a significant weight loss or call it an advantage. However, it is best to think of it as an excellent way to start your weight loss journey and lose a significant amount of weight at the beginning so that it motivates you to stay with the diet. So it is safe to say that losing water weight significantly helps in controlling weight gain and assists in managing weight.

High protein

Low carb diets are high in protein content and therefore an excellent option for those looking to develop lean muscles. Low protein foods such as sugars are replaced by high protein foods such as lean meats and seafood that help in developing stronger muscles.

Studies have shown that proteins tend to cut down on appetite and increase the rate of metabolism. It also helps in improving muscle mass in the body and replace fat cells. Metabolism helps in burning away calories thereby helping you maintain a lean frame.

Metabolism

Metabolism is an essential function of the body that helps in increasing fat burning capacity. Low carb diets are one of the best ways to increase your metabolism and lose weight rapidly. To put it simply, low carb diets will help you spend all your energy and lose weight quickly. The intake of lesser calories further helps in controlling weight gain and assists with the maintenance of a slim body. Various studies have found that a low carb diet helps in increasing energy levels and maintains the ideal body weight. The increase in metabolism is said to be around 250 calories, which are equal to an hour of exercise. So, it is best to increase the level of proteins in your diet so that you can enhance muscle growth. Apart from protein intake, there are other aspects of the diet that help with increasing muscle mass in the body. If the number of carbs is extremely low, then the glucose in the body begins to go through gluconeogenesis. This happens to be a repeated process and can help in burning away several calories. But this will only be a temporary phase, as the ketones will begin to replace the glucose that fuels the brain. The low carb diets have a metabolic advantage over the other diets and therefore must be considered first in case you wish to lose weight.

Lesser rewards

Low carb diets are highly recommended as they eliminate consumption of foods that are highly fattening. They do not promote junk and processed foods and eliminate everything that can add unnecessary fat to the body. These include the likes of aerated drinks, fruit juices with sugar, white, starchy bread, French fries, cakes, pizzas, etc. The diet also helps you eliminate high carb foods such as corn, wheat and sugar. This means that you deny your body all foods that can be fattening and calorific. Most of these foods come with high-calorie content, and you will not know how much is being consumed. The diet makes sure that this does not happen and you consume just the right amount of calories.

Appetite reduction

Low carb diets help in reducing the appetite significantly. Low carb diets are known to help in curbing the amount of food that you consume. This means that you do not binge on food and end up consuming more than what is required by your body. As soon as you adopt the diet, your appetite automatically goes down. This does not mean that the diet will make you starve; it just means that your appetite will go down, but you will eat until you feel full. The high protein content ensures that you do not suffer from hunger pangs and can feel full until the next meal. As you know, the level of ketones in your bloodstream will rise therefore making it easier for your body to burn away the fat easily. This will make you go for just 1 or 2 meals per day and feel full. There is also some proof that low carb diets help in regulating hunger hormones such as leptin and ghrelin. You will feel less hungry and full between meals.

Consistency

There have been reports that people who do not stick with the diet for long end up gaining back all the weight that they lost. It is therefore essential to maintain consistency and stick with the diet for more extended periods of time. Many people tend to take up the diet enthusiastically and end up abandoning it halfway through. This will only lead to excessive weight gain and an inability to lose the gained weight.

As you can see, the low carb diet works in many ways to help you develop a lean and slim body.

Women Specific Low Carb Diet

Carbohydrates tend to play an important role in weight loss, maintaining energy, recovering from exercises, balancing out your hormones, etc. Women's needs for carbs are different from what men need, and therefore, it is essential to consume the right amount of carbs per day. Some women tend to go on a low carb plan and include just 100 to 200 carbs in their diet per day, and some go even lower. Before you choose the number of calories, you have to make sure that you calculate your calorie intake and select the right amount.

Low carb diet for women

As mentioned earlier, the number of carbs that a woman consumes vary depending on her age, body type, physical activities, etc. Moderate to low carb diets will call for the consumption of 100 to 150 grams of carbs per day. This means you can consume about half cup of grains or a cup of dairy during meals along with a bowl of fresh fruits. Some low carb diets will make you limit the carb intake to just 50 grams per day or lesser. You will be asked to count the net carbs when you choose such diets. Net carbs include those that are digested by your body and affect your blood sugar levels. To find the net carbs in your diet, you must subtract the fiber in grams from the total carbs.

Women usually find it tough to know how many carbs they can consume to remain healthy as well as continue with the diet. Although all low carb diets will help in regularizing blood pressure and sugar levels, the number of carbs to be consumed varies from woman to woman.

Many factors need to be considered such as how active your lifestyle is, how fast or slow you recover from workouts if you have a thyroid issue, how regular or irregular are your periods, etc. It will be best to consult a nutritionist first to know how many calories you have to consume. Remember that this is especially important if you are pregnant or lactating.

Low carb diets

Most low carb plans will ask you to consume animal-based meats and leafy green vegetables. These will be filling and provide your body with the necessary nutrients. Women who are consuming between 100 to 200 grams of carbs can consume half a cup of whole grains; this can include quinoa and brown rice. You can also consume dairy products with some fruits.

Consume eggs on a daily basis and will be best for breakfast. You can consume it with cheddar cheese and an avocado along with a bowl of fruit such as papaya. The net carb will come up to 10. As for lunch, you can consume a bowl of vegetables along with some roasted chicken and fresh fruit such as apple and comes up to 20 grams. For dinner, you can consume a steak along with a cup of kale and a cup of brown rice that comes up to 46 net carbs. You can snack on quarter cup nuts such as almonds and drink a cup of low-fat milk, which comes to 24 and 14 grams each.

If you are going for 150 grams of carbs a day, then add a cup of oats in the morning and consume another fruit during lunchtime. If you wish to consume 50 to 100 grams, then forgo the fruit in the morning and remove the glass of milk. You can consume half a cup of brown rice for dinner.

Restrictive Diets

Remember that it is easier to lose weight during the first few stages of adopting a diet but becomes tougher as you progress. For this, you can take up very restrictive low-carb diets that limit you to no more than 50 grams of net carbs a day and can also go down to 20 in some cases. This type of diet is adapted to force your body to enter a state of ketosis so that your body produces ketones to provide energy. A ketogenic diet is known to help your body burn fat at a rapid pace and provide lasting results. However, the ketogenic diet is not suitable for all as it can be a bit tough on some women's bodies. You have to consult a physician before restricting the number of calories that you take in.

A restrictive low carb diet will make you consume more fat than your body is used to consuming. Your breakfast will be made of bacon and eggs. During lunch, you can consume lean chicken curry with cottage cheese and a simple cucumber salad. For dinner, you can consume beef stir-fry, a bowl of water-rich vegetables and snack on a hard-boiled egg.

Low carb diet needs
Women require lots of calcium and iron when they take up a diet. These two are not easy for the body to synthesize from food that is consumed. Good sources of these include milk, yogurt and grains. However, these are not allowed as per a strict low carb diet thereby denying your body some of these nutrients. You can consume nuts, low-fat dairy such as milk, Greek yogurt and cheeses. However, you have to limit it to no more than 20 grams per day. Kale and salmon with their bones in also give you a good dose of calcium. If you think the calcium level in your body is quite low then consume a calcium supplement

Iron is an essential component that helps in keeping red blood cells healthy. You can incorporate red meats in your diet to meet the iron requirement. This is especially important for women who are going through menopause and would like to counter the blood loss. Spinach is a very rich source of iron and should be consumed regularly. Sardines can also provide you with the required amount of iron.

Some low carb diets can interfere with the production hormones and will therefore not be ideal for some women. Eating too little carbs can sometimes cause hormonal imbalance and lead to irregular periods. This can lead to a condition known as amenorrhea.

Low carb diets can also interfere with thyroid function. It can reverse T3 and cause it to decrease in the body. RT3 can go up and result in poor metabolism, lower concentration and lead to irritation. You have to give your health primary importance and ensure that you pay attention to these signs and symptoms and avoid falling prey to adverse effects of the diet.

Low Carb Tips for Women

Here are some low carb tips that women can follow.

Protein intake

Regularizing the protein intake is important. It is understood that the low carb diet is a high protein diet. This does not mean that you consume too much protein. Women require lesser protein compared to men and can easily manage to get the daily requirement through smart meal planning. Some women end up over-consuming protein that can lead to issues such as loose motions and flatulence. If you and your husband happen to be eating the same portions of meals such as meats, then you will be over consuming proteins.

Too much protein can also lead to a dysfunction in ketosis. Your body might not be able to burn fat rapidly. After a protein-rich meal, check your blood sugar levels to see if they are spiked up. If it does, then some of the protein you consumed has been turned to sugar. This will, in turn, slow down your bodily processes.

It is advisable for women to consume between 0.5 and 1.5 grams of protein per body weight. Therefore, a person weighing 155 lbs should consume about 105 grams of protein a day or lesser if possible.

Proteins tend to make you feel full. So many women end up consuming more just to be able to limit their meals to 2 per day. This is not the right approach to adopt. It is especially important for menopausal women to maintain the correct level of proteins in their diet. It might take a little time for you to retrain your body and get it to accept lesser proteins and remain full between meals.

Go about the process in a systematic manner and give your body enough time to get adjusted to the diet. Most women are advised to give it at least one week so that the diet settles in and their bodies can accept it. Experts advise that women engage in mindful eating. This is a technique where people mindfully cut down on the amount of protein intake for some time. For example, if you are used to consuming two eggs for breakfast then cut it down to one egg for a week. You will see that it is helping your diet.

After consuming a meal, that has lesser protein than what your systems are used to- but meets your daily requirement, you have to wait for 5 minutes to see if you are still hungry. If you happen to be hungry, then eat a little more, but if you feel like you have had enough, then you can stop. It is always better than saying I had too much or I could have avoided eating an extra egg.

Control fat intake

It is understood that a low carb diet is all about consuming more fat and lesser carbs. However, this does not mean you end up overeating fat. Once you start out by eating more fat and accustoming your body to it, you have to cut down on it gradually. Remember that it is still a diet and you have to burn away your existing fat to develop a slim body. The best way to do this is by ensuring that you eat just the right amount of fat that will help with the production of ketones. You have to measure out the amount of fat you are consuming so that it is easier for your body to adapt to it. If you are used to adding butter to your coffee, then you should cut down on it. Similarly, stop consuming fat bombs and try to control your fat intake for a week.

The best way to go about this is by gradually cutting down on the fat you consume. Give yourself a week's time and go about it slowly so that your body adjusts to it. Once you enter the state of ketosis, you can slow down on the fat consumption and can even stop.

Some people complain that their weight is not reducing despite taking on the diet. In such a case, it is best to revaluate the diet and try to cut back as much as possible on the fat content. Come up with dishes that are tasty and well seasoned and will not make you miss the fat. But remember that this does not mean you starve yourself. You have to consume a little fat and eat healthy meals that will help you develop a fit body.

One place where many people go wrong is they over-consume fats in the form of liquids. Whipping cream is a source of fat that most people tend to ignore and end up over consuming. Similarly, you have to cut back on stocks and broths that are full of fat. They can interfere with your weight loss and prevent you from experiencing positive results. Once you reach your goal or ideal weight, then you can add the fat back to the diet.

Intermittent fasts

Once your body adapts to the fat, you can take up intermittent fasting. This fast is simple and can be carried out for more extended periods of time. Once your body is fat adapted your body will get used to the process of ketosis and lead to a diminished appetite. People stop consuming breakfast and go straight to lunch and dinner. This is done on purpose so that they can fast for 16 hours. They consume their first meal 5 to 6 hours after waking up. Try the fast out by first dieting for 10 hours and then gradually stretch it to 16 hours. Next, you have to eat lunch and dinner within an 8-hour window. The fast is known as a 16:8 fast. You can also try out the 24-hour fast where you eat dinner one night and wait until the next night to eat dinner.

As per study reports, intermittent fasting has helped people lose stubborn fat such as visceral fat that is around the stomach area. The idea is to adopt a fast that fits well into your eating and lifestyle routine. You can always switch up the routine and not stick with just one. For example, you can take up the 16:8 one day and the 24 hour-fast another day and so on. Stick with the one that works best for your body.

You should eat when you are hungry and stop as soon as you feel full. Drink a tall glass of water as soon as you go halfway through your meal so that you feel full and give your body the chance to digest the meal better. But remember that you have to listen to your body and pay attention to the hunger signs so that you eat when your body needs food.

Sides

Pay attention to side dishes. Many sides such as sauces, condiments and snacks can add back unnecessary carbs. You have to avoid these as much as possible and ensure that you only eat healthy foods. You can prepare your sauces and condiments at home. Make use of fresh, natural ingredients so that you make tasty, healthy condiments.

Remove alcohol

Remove alcohol from your diet. The low carb diet does not encourage consumption of alcohol. This applies to hard liquor. You can have an occasional glass of wine but must limit it to just two glasses a month. If you start consuming alcohol then as soon as you start experiencing weight loss then you will end up negating it and start gaining again. Remember that just a few drinks are enough to reverse the positive effects of the diet and so, it is a must to not engage in drinking activities while on the diet. If you have an addiction, then consider visiting rehab so that you can defeat the habit and develop a healthier body.

Smoking/drugs

Smoking and consuming recreational drugs can both negatively impact your health. They will release more cortisol in your brain and interfere with regular bodily function. In such a case it is best to avoid engaging in these and focusing on healthier habits.

Do not consume sweeteners

Avoid consuming sweeteners as much as possible. Artificial sweeteners contain aspartame, which is said to be a sweet compound found in certain plants. Although they will replace the sugar in your diet they will not do much regarding losing weight. As per studies, people who cut out artificial sweeteners from their diet were able to lose weight faster.

Aerobic exercises

Exercising should be taken up to promote weight loss. There are many types to choose from such as cycling, skipping, swimming, etc. These are known as aerobic exercises and involve getting the heart rate up. Once your heart rate is up, it will lead to greater weight loss. Try out one exercise each week and stick with the one that helps you most. Don't forget to warm up for 15 minutes before taking up an exercise.

Anaerobic exercises

You have to take up anaerobic exercises to develop a lean body. Some of them include lifting weights, doing lunges, mountain climbing, etc. Do these for at least 15 minutes every day so that your body feels worked. These exercises work better for weight loss compared to aerobic exercises. Those are meant to get your heart rate up while these help in toning down the muscles and replacing fat cells with lean muscles.

You don't have to lift heavy weights and can limit it to whatever you are comfortable with. Work with a fitness trainer to learn what the ideal weight is that you can lift. Don't lift weights for too long or on a day-to-day basis. You can lift them every alternate day. Remember that your muscles will tell you when to stop and when they need more. If it starts to tingle, then you must carry on, but it starts to tighten and begins to hurt then you have to stop.

Remember that exercise is not paramount for weight loss. Yes, it is essential as it helps in fastening the process of weight loss and developing lean muscles. However, you must focus first on your diet and then on exercise.

If you engage in too much exercise, then it can lead to a false weight loss. You will feel like you have lost quite a bit of weight, but in reality, you would have only lost some water weight. This weight will be back within a couple of weeks. Too much exercise can also lead to soreness and muscle inflammation, which is not healthy.

Take at least two days break so that your body can recover from the exercise routine.

Sleep well

You must get a good night's sleep if you wish to develop a lean body and healthy mind. Make sure you get at least eight straight hours of sleep per night. Most women end up staying up late into the night and negatively impacting their health. You must avoid engaging in distractions such as watching television. You can meditate before going to bed so that your mind is free from thoughts.

Here are a few tips that you can try out to sleep better.

- Make sure the room is dark and cool. The ideal temperature should be 20 degrees, and there should be just 5% light coming in. There should be no blue light as it can disrupt sleep. You can wear eye masks if there is too much light
- Playing a light music can help you sleep better. White noise such as the sound of waterfalls can help you sleep faster
- Make it a point to go to bed at the same time every day even on weekends
- Expose yourself to natural sunlight every day
- You should maintain a hygienic bedroom to get a good night's sleep

Control stress

You should control stress as much as possible. Stress can negatively impact your health and make it difficult for you to carry on with the diet. In fact, it can negate the effects of the diet and make it difficult for you to get the results.

36

Stress causes your body to release a chemical known as cortisol. This chemical can interfere with regular bodily function. It is especially important for women of a menopausal age not to stress out and maintain a cool and collected mind. Many things in life can get the best of you such as children moving out, stress of retirement, etc. You must make an effort not to let these affect you.

There are many simple techniques that you can try out to put an end to stress. Some of them include taking up yoga, exercising, Pilates, pursuing a hobby, etc. Do whatever distracts you and keeps you calm.

Excessive stress can lead to emotional eating as well. This can lead to unnecessary weight gain. You can indulge in a technique known as mindfulness. As per this method, you focus on the task at hand and cut out the rest of the world. For example, you switch on some music and focus on it. This will distract you and take your mind off a stressful situation and can also distract you from indulging in your cravings.

Expectations
As a rule, you must set realistic expectations and make sure that you do not pressure yourself to achieve something that is tough to attain. This tip is especially important for women to follow as they tend to pressurize themselves to see faster results and are often let down. Some women tend to set a weight loss number that is not practical or healthy and give into the pressure of other people advising them to attain an ideal weight that is not practical.

Remember that you are taking on the low carb diet not because you wish to lose weight and develop a lean body but because you wish to protect your body from illness and lead a longer life. So do not measure the success of the diet regarding the number of kilograms you lose but instead about the number of health benefits that you received from the diet.

Remember that your body fat percentage should be measured to check whether you have experienced any significant loss. Measure it every few months so that you know how the diet is going.

Supplements and Nutrients

Just switching to a low carb diet will not give you the results you want to see. You will have to bring about a lifestyle change, which includes ensuring that you consume certain nutrients and supplements in your diet. Some of these are a part of the meal you consume, while others have to be externally consumed. It is best to consult your physician before you take any extra supplements.

Here are some nutrients and supplements to add to your diet.

Electrolytes
It can be a little difficult for your body to get the right salts and other nutrients through diet alone and so, you must consume an electrolyte to add back some of the lost salts. If these remain depleted, then you can suffer from headaches, nausea and fatigue. As carbohydrates are removed from your diet, so are electrolytes such as sodium and potassium. You should consume an electrolyte that will add these back to your body. If you experience dehydration, then make sure you drink more electrolytes and take a little rest to help your body recover.

Coconut oil
You have to add coconut oil to your diet. It is known that nuts and seeds such as almonds and peanuts help in providing your body with the required amounts of proteins, calories and carbs. However, they can be a little fattening and so, you have to ensure that you incorporate an ingredient that is low in fat and high in nutrition. MCT or coconut oil happens to be one such ingredient that you can use to get the daily requirement of carbs. MCT stands for medium chain triglycerides and gives your body 14 grams of fat in every tablespoon. You can add coconut and MCT oil in all your meals such as curries and soups. You can also add a tablespoon of it to your coffee. It has a high heating

point and so can be used in cooking. Add a little to your milkshakes and smoothies as well.

Fiber

Fiber is an essential ingredient to incorporate into your diet if you wish to lose weight. Fiber is something that your body cannot digest. However, it fools the body into thinking that it can digest it and forces it to put in a lot more energy. This helps in burning fat. There are many sources of natural fiber such as beans, green leafy vegetables, fruits such as papaya, etc. Try to have at least one bowl of these with each meal. You can also consume a fiber-rich powder that will add back the necessary fiber to your body. One advantage of consuming fiber is that it helps you feel full and avoid hunger pangs.

Caffeine

Caffeine can help you lose weight faster. Having a cup of coffee with a dollop of butter before working out and one after working out can help you develop a lean and slim body. The rate at which your body burns fat will be enhanced. You can burn away more fat within a short amount of time. Do not add any sugar or sweetener though.

Greens

Greens and green leafy vegetables are one of the most essential ingredients required to develop a lean and healthy body. Most of us end up not getting enough of these ingredients, as our diets do not incorporate them. In such a case, we have to make the effort of adding them to our diet or consuming a supplement that contains the same nutrients. Make a conscious effort to get more greens into your diet. Choose green ones such as cruciferous vegetables. Add a handful of spinach to all your meals including breakfast, lunch and dinner. Make smoothies using green vegetables and leafy greens. Ask your doctor about a supplement that can replace the nutrients in your diet.

Ashwagandha

Ashwagandha is an herb that helps in controlling the cortisol levels in your brain. This helps in increasing the diet's positive effects on the body. The herb also helps in enhancing brain function and heart function. You can consume it in the form of tablets, powder or syrup. But you might have to consult a physician first to check whether it is safe to consume this supplement.

Ginseng

Ginseng is a natural herb that has been used in China for several centuries. It is used to combat weight gain and develop a lean and healthy body. Ginseng is a potent herb that can efficiently replace the fat cells in your body. The herb is also used to combat some of the side effects associated with low carb diets such as fatigue and dehydration. You can consume it in tablet and powder form.

Curcumin

Curcumin is a naturally occurring compound that is found in turmeric and ginger. This compound helps in cutting down on the fat cells in your body. According to studies, turmeric helps in controlling the development and growth of fat tissues in your body. It helps in increasing immunity. It is full of antioxidants that help in keeping your cells healthy. Curcumin is also an anti-inflammatory and helps in controlling the onset of illnesses such as common cold. You can add just a little to your curries, soups and sprinkle it over salads. Speak with your doctor to know whether you have to take any other supplement to develop and maintain a healthy body.

Low Carb Breakfast Recipes

Here are some tasty low-carb breakfast recipes.

Almond and Flaxseed Pancakes

Yields 6 servings

Ingredients

½ teaspoon salt

330g almond flour

½ teaspoon baking soda

3 eggs

1 tablespoon ground flaxseed

1 tablespoon butter

180ml unsweetened almond milk

Directions

1. Mix the flaxseeds, baking soda, salt, and almond flour in a bowl.

2. Whisk the eggs in another bowl.

3. Add butter and milk to the eggs and mix the mixture thoroughly.

4. Whisk in the flour mixture into the egg mixture gradually. You can add more milk if required, one tablespoon at a time. Mix everything well together.

5. On moderate heat, heat a frying pan and add oil to it.

6. Pour about four tablespoons of the pancake batter onto it and cook each side for about three minutes. Repeat this step with the remaining batter until you get about six pancakes. Serve and enjoy.

Each pancake contains 12.9g fat, 7.6g protein, and 1.2g net carbs.

Almond Biscotti

Yields 10 servings

Ingredients

2 teaspoons Splenda

½ teaspoon baking powder

2 eggs

1 tablespoon ground almonds

½ teaspoon vanilla extract

½ teaspoon almond extract

½ teaspoon salt

80g almond flour

4 tablespoons butter

Directions

1. Preheat the oven. Line a baking sheet using parchment paper. Grease it lightly.

2. Mix almonds, almond flour, butter, salt and baking powder in a bowl.. Add the extracts, Splenda, and eggs to the dry mixture and mix all the ingredients well. Leave the batter for about five minutes, for the almond meal to absorb any leftover liquid.

3. When the dough becomes firm, but soft, place it onto your baking sheet and create a rectangle of it.

4. Bake it until its top gets a light brown hue. This will roughly take around 25 minutes.

5. Take it out of the oven and let it cool. Cut slices of it and serve.

Each biscotti contains 07.g carbs, 2.1g protein, and 5.8g fat.

Almond Berry Smoothie

Yields 1 serving

Ingredients

150g raspberries

300ml unsweetened almond milk

4 tablespoons whipped cream

1 scoop unsweetened soya protein powder

25 almonds

Directions

1. Add all the ingredients excluding the whipped cream to the blender and blend until you achieve your desired consistency.

2. Pour the smoothie into a glass and top it with whipped cream. Serve and enjoy.

This smoothie contains 11.7g net carbs, 22.9g protein, and 29.1g fat.

Greek Salad Omelette

Yields 4- 6 servings

Ingredients

10 eggs

2 tablespoons olive oil

A handful of parsley leaves (chopped)

1 large red onion (cut into wedges)

Large handful of black olives

3 tomatoes (chopped into chunks)

100g feta cheese (crumbled)

Directions

1. Heat your grill to high.

2. Break the eggs in a bowl and whisk them along with chopped parsley, salt and pepper if you wish.

3. Heat oil in a non stick pan over high heat and fry onion wedges for around four minutes, until their edges begin to brown.

4. Add in the olives and tomatoes and cook them for two minutes, or until they become tender.

5. Reduce the heat to medium. Add in the beaten eggs. Cook the eggs and stir them as they set until they are half-set. Sprinkle the feta cheese on top and place the frying pan in the grill for five to six minutes until the omelet becomes golden and puffed up. Cut it into wedges and serve.

Each serving contains 5g net carbs, 24g protein, and 28g fat.

Asparagus Frittata

Yields 4 servings

Ingredients

115g brie

1 teaspoon black pepper

1 teaspoon salt

1 garlic clove

8 eggs

4 tablespoons extra-virgin olive oil

8 asparagus

Directions

1. Preheat your oven to about 232 degrees Centigrade or the gas mark 8.

2. Trim the asparagus ends. Cut each piece into 5mm slices.

3. Heat oil in a frying pan over moderate heat and add the asparagus to the pan. Fry it for about three to four minutes.

4. Add garlic to the asparagus and cook it for about one minute.

5. Add pepper, salt and eggs to a bowl and mix the ingredients well. Add this mixture to the pan and reduce the heat to low. Cook it until the edges begin to set.

6. Use a rubber spatula to lift the frittata while tilting your pan. The uncooked side of the egg should flow underneath, so it gets cooked. Let it cook for about one to two minutes. You can put some shredded cheese on top (this is optional.)

7. Put the pan in the oven for about seven to ten minutes. Take it out and serve.

Each serving contains 0.9g net carbs, 20.6g protein, and 32.2g fat.

Asparagus and Cheese

Yields 1 serving

Ingredients

2 eggs

2 bacon slices

30g cheddar cheese

6 asparagus

Directions

1. Cook the bacon slices in a pan. Save some of the fat.

2. Chop the bacon into tiny pieces.

3. Cook the asparagus sticks separately in the reserved bacon fat. Cook them for around three minutes. Remove from the heat and cut them into small, bite-sized pieces.

4. Put all the ingredients in the pan once again. This time, add the egg. Scramble everything and cook until the egg is properly cooked and the cheese starts to melt. This takes roughly three minutes. Serve and enjoy.

Each serving contains 2.8g net carbs, 23.2g fat, and 27.4g protein.

Keto Bagel

Yields 6 bagels

Ingredients

1 tablespoon of baking powder

1 teaspoon of Celtic sea salt

6 egg whites

½ cup of pumpkin seeds

½ cup of hemp hearts

½ cup of sesame seeds

¼ cup of Psyllium Fiber

1 cup of coconut flour

Directions

1. Preheat your oven to 350 degrees F.

2. Mix all the dry ingredients in a large mixing bowl.

3. Whisk the egg whites until they appear foamy.

4. Pour the beaten egg whites into the bowl with the dry ingredients and use a spoon to mix. You are supposed to end up with crumbly dough.

5. Add in 1 cup of boiling water. Stir until you have smooth dough that can stick together but is still a little bit crumbly.

6. Lay down a piece of parchment paper on a cookie sheet.

7. Create 6 dough balls from the huge dough. Hold the ball in one hand and then make a hole in the dough. You can do this by sticking your thumb through it.

8. Lay down the dough on the cookie sheet and start forming it into a bagel by using your fingers to press it together.

9. Sprinkle the dough with some poppy seeds or sesame seeds.

10. Place the dough on the cookie sheet in the oven and cook for about 55 minutes at 350 degrees F.

11. Once done, let it cool for a couple of minutes in the oven. That will give it an extra crunchy top.

Serve and enjoy.

Each serving contains 19g fat, 8g net carbs, 18g protein.

Cheese Omelets with Fresh Salsa

Yields 2 servings

Ingredients

1 cup of shredded Monterey Jack cheese

1 tablespoon of unsalted butter

3 medium slices of bacon

4 large eggs

1 tablespoon of fresh lime juice

1 oz. of cilantro

½ Jalapeno peppers

3 medium spring or scallion onions

1 medium sized tomato

Directions

1. First prepare the salsa. Finely chop the jalapeno, tomatoes and green onions and place them in a small sized mixing bowl. Add in lime juice and cilantro, and then use a spoon to mix. Season with salt and pepper to taste and set aside.

2. Whisk the eggs with water in a separate mixing bowl.

3. Prepare the bacon by cooking it thoroughly. Crumble the bacon and set aside.

4. Place a small nonstick skillet over medium-high heat.

5. Melt half the butter and wait until the foam subsides. Once it does, add in half the egg mixture as you tilt the pan to coat the whole surface. Cook for about 1 minute.

6. Add in cheese, sliced avocado and half the crumbled bacon and cook for another 1 minute.

7. Transfer to a plate and serve with salsa.

Each Serving Contains 33g Protein, 42.5g Fats and 3.9g Net Carbs.

Green Buttered Eggs

Yields 2 Servings

Ingredients

4 organic eggs

½ cup fresh parsley, chopped

½ cup fresh cilantro, chopped

½ teaspoon sea salt

1 teaspoon thyme leaves, fresh

2 garlic cloves, finely chopped

1 tablespoon coconut oil

2 tablespoon organic butter

¼ teaspoon cayenne, ground

¼ teaspoon cumin, ground

Directions

1. Melt butter and coconut oil in a non-stick skillet for 60 seconds.

2. Add chopped garlic and cook for 3 minutes on a low flame. Once the garlic begins to brown, add thyme.

3. Brown for 30-60 seconds then add in parsley and cilantro. Cook until the thyme begins to crisp on moderate flame.

4. After around 3 minutes, add eggs in the pan. Crack them straight in without breaking the yolk.

5. Cover the pan, set the heat to low and cook for 4-6 minutes. Once the yolks are set; serve.

Each serving contains 27.5g *Fat, 2.5g Carbs and 12.8g Protein*

Low-Carb Lunch Recipes

Here are some mouth-watering, low carb lunch recipes for you to enjoy.

Antipasti Skewers

Yields 8 servings

Ingredients

1 bell pepper

8 slices of prosciutto

8 cherry tomatoes

8 kalamata olives

100g courgette

4 servings of salami genoa

8 mushrooms

1 tablespoon olive oil

1 tablespoon balsamic vinegar

1 tablespoon lemon juice

1 teaspoon dried oregano

1 garlic clove

1 teaspoon ground pepper

1 teaspoon salt

Directions

1. Soak bamboo skewers in water for around 15 minutes.

2. Cut the bell pepper into slices and wrap one porscuitto slice around one slice of bell pepper.

3. Thread every skewer with one tomato, one olive, one cube of courgette, one mushroom, one prosciutto wrapped pepper, and one salami cube.

4. Put the skewers in a baking dish, preferably a shallow one.

5. Put lemon juice, garlic, oregano, oil, vinegar, pepper and salt in a bowl and mix them well. Pour this mixture over the skewers and coat them well.

6. Preheat your grill and grill the skewers until the veggies become tender. This takes about four to five minutes.

Each skewer contains 2.6g net carbs, 11.9g protein, and 10.4g fat.

Paillard of Chicken with Herbs and Lemon

Yields 6 servings

Ingredients

2 tablespoons olive oil

6 skinless chicken breasts

½ tablespoon balsamic vinegar

25g Parmesan cheese

140g bag rocket leaves

Lemon wedges

For the marinade

3 rosemary sprigs (leaves should be chopped)

2 garlic cloves

Zest of 1 lemon

6 sage leaves (finely shredded)

3 tablespoons olive oil

Juice of ½ lemon

Directions

1. Place every chicken breast between two sheets of baking parchment paper or cling film. Bash every piece with a rolling pin. Flatten it out to a 0.5cm thick layer and then put it in a dish.

2. Crush the garlic cloves using mortar and pestle. Add one pinch salt to it. Add sage and rosemary and pound all the ingredients well together. Add in the lemon juice and lemon zest followed by ground black pepper and olive oil. This is your marinade. Pour it over the chicken breasts and coat the breasts well in it. Cover them and chill them for a minimum of two hours.

4. Heat your barbecue. When the flames diminish, spread coals in it evenly. Cook chicken in it, one to two minutes on both the sides. Transfer the pieces to a board. Leave them for a couple of minutes.

5. Meanwhile, add balsamic vinegar and oil in a bowl and add in the rocket leaves along with some seasoning. Toss them well and sprinkle Parmesan on top. Serve it with the chicken and lemon wedges.

Each serving contains 1g net carbs, 12g fat, and 32g protein.

Tuna Salad

Yields 1 serving

Ingredients

3 Bok Choy

175g tuna fillet

6 radishes

30g tinned water chestnuts

1 tablespoon soya sauce

1 tomato

Directions

1. Grill the tuna fillets.

2. Steam the Bok Choy.

3. Stir fry the remaining ingredients in soya sauce and then put the Bok Choy, tuna fillets and fried veggies on a plate. Enjoy.

Each serving contains 6.1g net carbs, 72.4g protein, and 14.2g fat.

Aubergine Melts

Yields 4 servings

Ingredients

2 aubergines (halved lengthways)

3 tablespoons olive oil

4 tomatoes

Handful of basil leaves

150g mozzarella ball (drained)

Directions

1. Heat the oven to gas mark 6, or 200 degrees Centigrade.

2. Drizzle oil over the cut aubergine. Bake them for about 25 minutes, or until they become tender.

3. Slice tomatoes and cheese, and arrange them on the top of the baked aubergine.

4. Put them in the oven for five more minutes, or until the cheese starts to melt. Scatter some basil leaves on top and serve.

Each aubergine melt contains 7g net carbs, 9g protein, and 17g fat.

Fennel and Prawn Salad

Makes 4 servings

Ingredients

2 tablespoons lemon juice

4 tablespoons olive oil

50g fennel

200g large prawns

1 avocado

100g rocket leaves

3 spring onions

Salt and pepper to taste

Directions

1. Mix the lemon juice and oil in a bowl and season it with pepper and salt. This will be your salad's dressing.

2. Toss the rest of the ingredients in another bowl, excluding rocket leaves. Pour half of the salad dressing and mix well.

3. Scatter rocket leaves into the serving bowls and put the salad at the centre. Drizzle the leftover dressing on the top before you serve the salad.

Each serving contains 2.8g net carbs, 18.2g protein, and 20.1g fat.

Pork Chops

Yields 3 servings

Ingredients

1 tablespoon of balsamic vinegar

1 cup of mayonnaise

1 teaspoon of ground nutmeg

1 teaspoon of garlic powder

3 medium sized boneless pork chops

½ cup of oil

1 package of washed sliced brown mushrooms

1 medium sized yellow onion, peeled and sliced

Directions

1. Preheat the oven to 350 degrees F.

2. Sauté the onions and mushrooms in a large skillet with some oil.

3. Push the onions and mushrooms to the side in order to make some space for the pork chops.

3. Add in the pork chops and season the pork chops with nutmeg and garlic powder. Brown the pork chops on each side.

4. Transfer the pork chop skillet into the oven and let it cook for 30 minutes or until the chops record at least 165 degree F on the meat thermometer.

5. Remove the skillet from the oven and place it on the stovetop. Transfer the pork chops to a plate and set aside.

6. Pour in vinegar and mayo to the oil and onions that were left on the pan. Whisk the mixture until well combined. You should end up with a thick sauce.

7. Pour the sauce over the chops in the plate. Serve and enjoy.

Each serving contains 103 g fats, 8g net carbs, 30g protein.

Turkey Burger

Yields 4 servings

Ingredients

½ bunch of finely chopped cilantro leaves

8 ounce can water chestnuts, drained and coarsely chopped

1-inch piece of grated and peeled ginger

1 tablespoon of sambal oelek

¼ cup of soy sauce

1 ½ pounds of ground turkey

2 smashed and finely chopped garlic clove

Kosher salt to taste

1 onion, cut into ¼ inch slices

Extra virgin olive oil

Others

Butter lettuce

4 slices of raw red onion

4 slices of beefsteak tomatoes

¼ cup of mayo that has 2 teaspoon mixture of sambal oelek

4 burger buns

4 slices of cheddar

Directions

1. Start by preheating the oven to 200 degrees.

2. Coat a large pan with some olive oil and place it over medium high heat. Add in the onions and cook them for 7-8 minutes or until soft; season with salt.

3. Add in garlic and cook for a further 1 or 2 minutes. Turn off the heat and let this cool down.

4. Place the cooked garlic and onion in a large mixing bowl (don't wash the sauté pan as you will use it later on). Add in cilantro, water chestnuts, ginger, sambal oelek, soy sauce, ½ cup of water and turkey. Combine everything together using your hands; season the patty to your liking. Use your hands to form four equal sized patties.

5. Coat the sauté pan that you used to cook onions with olive oil and place over medium-high heat.

6. Place the patties in the pan and cook them for 5-6 minutes each side. If your pan is small, you can work in batches of 2 patties to avoid crowding the pan. Add in cheese and cook for 1 more minute.

7. Toast your buns in a toaster or a broiler. Lightly apply both sides of the bun with sambaal mayo.

8. Place a burger on the bottom bun and top it with lettuce, onion and tomato, and then place the top bun. Serve and enjoy.

Each serving contains 6g fats, 0.68g net carbs and 44g protein.

Keto Cobb Salad

Yields 2 Servings

Ingredients

2 slices of turkey bacon

½ avocado diced

2 cups of romaine lettuce, coarsely chopped

2 hard-boiled eggs

30g of blue cheese

4 cherry tomatoes

100g of Ham

2-3 tablespoons olive oil cooking spray, extra virgin

For the dressing:

Pinch of garlic

Salt and pepper to taste

1 teaspoon of Dijon Mustard

1 teaspoon of lemon juice

1 tablespoon of apple cider vinegar, organic

1 tablespoons of olive oil

Directions

1. Prepare hard boiled eggs through regular method or by a pre-programmed steam process.

2. Then slice the ham in cubes. Spray a non-stick skillet with olive oil and heat the sliced ham for about 3-5 minutes.

3. Slice the hard boiled eggs and then position the lettuce onto the bottom the bowl.

4. Arrange the turkey bacon, ham, eggs, blue cheese, avocados and cherry tomatoes in rows next to each other.

5. Then spread the dressing over the mixture. If desired, you can reduce the amount of tomatoes to further reduce carb intake.

Each serving contains 27g Fat, 7g Carb and 46g Proteins

Low-Carb Dinner Recipes

Let us share some delicious and nutritious low-carb dinner recipes with you now.

Carbonara Penne

Yields 1 serving

Ingredients

2 tablespoons parmesan cheese

25g Atkins penne pasta

1 teaspoon fresh parsley

1 teaspoon black pepper

1 teaspoon salt

½ garlic clove

1 egg

30ml single cream

2 bacon slices

Directions

1. Boil the penne. Cook until al dente. Remove from the heat and drain it well.

2. Cut the bacon into thin strips. Fry them until they get a golden brown hue.

3. Crush the garlic clove and add it to the bacon followed by parsley. Cook them for a couple of seconds, and then remove the bacon strips from the heat.

4. Put the drained penne in the frying pan and cook it. Add all the other ingredients to it including the bacon and the egg. Add only about half of the grated cheese. Season it using pepper and salt.

5. Serve and sprinkle the remaining cheese on top.

Each serving contains 7.8g net carbs, 30.9g protein, and 18.9g fat.

Lamb Shashlik with Rosemary

Yields 14 skewers

Ingredients

1 lemon, juiced and roughly chopped

1 1 ½ kg lamb leg, boned and cut into big chunks

3 tablespoons olive oil

Handful of rosemary springs, picked and chopped

20 garlic cloves, finely chopped

2 red onions, cut into wedges

3 cubed green peppers

To Serve

Natural yogurt

Warmed flatbreads

Chopped cucumber and tomato

Chili sauce

Directions

1. Put lamb, oil, rosemary, garlic, lemon juice, and lemon in a bowl and mix. Season well and then cover it using cling film. Chill it for a couple of hours.

2. Thread the pieces of lamb on wooden skewers; alternate them with onions and peppers.

3. Heat the coals on the barbecue and put the lamb skewers on them. Cook for about five minutes, or until they get a nice colour. Turn and cook the other side for another five to ten minutes, until they become nicely charred. To test the lamb, put a skewer in the middle of the lamb. If bloody juice runs from it, it is not properly cooked, but if the juice is watery and pink, the piece has been cooked. Keep the meat aside for a couple of

minutes before you serve them with the foods mentioned under the 'to serve' subheading.

Each serving contains 3g net carbs, 21g protein, and 16g fat.

Avocado Burger

Yields 1 serving

Ingredients

½ avocado

100g hamburger patty

1 tomato

50g mixed salad leaves

1 romaine leaf

Directions

1. Grill the hamburger patty.

2. Slice tomato and avocado and place them on the burger.

3. Serve it on a romaine leaf surrounded by mixed salad leaves. Enjoy!

Each serving contains 4.1g net carbs, 47.6g protein, and 29.6g fat.

Steamed Fish

Yields 4 servings

Ingredients

2 pak choi, thickly sliced

4 plaice haddock or any MSC-certified white fish fillet

4 spring onions, shredded

3cm ginger, cut in the form of matchsticks

Juice of 1 lime

2 tablespoon reduced salt soya sauce

1 red chili, thinly sliced

1 teaspoon sesame oil

Directions

1. Heat the oven to gas mark 6 or 200 degrees Centigrade.

2. Put each fish fillet in the middle of a big foil square. Top it with spring onions, ginger, chili, and pak choi. Pull up the foil's edges.

3. Mix lime juice, one tablespoon water and soya sauce in a bowl and then spoon a little on the top of every fillet. Enclose the fillets by crimping the foil's top.

4. Place these fish parcels on a baking sheet.

5. Bake for about 10 to 15 minutes, or until the fish is well cooked. Open the parcels, drizzle a little sesame oil on it and serve.

Each fillet contains 2g net carbs, 3g fat, and 22g protein.

Goan Mussels

Yields 4 servings

Ingredients

Sunflower oil to fry the mussels

1kg fresh mussel

1 chopped onion

1 piece of thumb-sized ginger, grated

2 chopped green chilies

4 crushed cloves of garlic

½ teaspoon ground turmeric

1 teaspoon black mustard seed

2 teaspoons ground coriander

2 teaspoons ground cumin

Coriander sprigs for serving

Lime wedges for serving

400ml coconut milk

Directions

1. Remove the mussel beards and wash them with cold water. Wash them in clean water several times until the water becomes clear. Discard any broken mussels, or those that stay open when you tap them.

2. Heat oil in a casserole, preferably flameproof one. Fry the onion until it gets a light brown hue. Add in garlic, ginger, spices, chilies, salt, and pepper and cook for about two to three minutes until they are well toasted.

3. Add in the coconut milk. Boil it and let it simmer for a couple of minutes.

4. Add in the mussels and increase the heat to very high. Boil for about three to four minutes or until the mussels open. Scatter coriander sprigs on them and serve with the lime wedges.

Each serving contains 9g net carbs, 14g protein and 23g fat.

Chicken Casserole

Yields 2 servings

Ingredients

2 tablespoons olive oil

100g courgette

2 cloves garlic

½ red onion

100g cauliflower

100g aubergine

½ red bell pepper

150ml chicken stock

200g peeled and canned tomatoes

4 chicken thighs with skin

2 teaspoons fresh parsley

5 black olives

Pepper and salt for seasoning

Directions

1. Put the chicken thighs in a pan and fry, and then set aside.

2. Heat the oven to about 200 degrees Centigrade and pour oil in a roasting tin.

3. Add in garlic and the veggies in it and coat them in the oil.

4. Place chicken thighs on the veggies and season them.

5. Roast for about 45 minutes.

6. Remove the garlic from the tin and squeeze its juice on the vegetables.

7. Simmer the tomatoes in a frying pan until they start to bubble. Add in the stock and season it.

8. Pour it over the roasted thighs and veggies. Put olives and parsley on top and serve.

Each serving contains 8.8g net carbs, 78.7g protein, and 66g fat.

Low-Carb Dessert Recipes

Here are scrumptious low-carb dessert recipes for you to satisfy your sweet tooth.

Ricotta Cheesecakes

Yields 4 servings

Ingredients

1 teaspoon vanilla extract

2 Splenda packets

2 egg whites

250g ricotta cheese

Raspberries

Directions

1. Break the ricotta cheese in a bowl.

2. Add vanilla extract, splenda and egg whites to it, and mix well.

3. Grease four ramekin dishes and spoon the cheesecake mixture equally into all the dishes.

4. Bake for 20 minutes in the oven at 176 degrees centigrade, or until the cheesecakes have properly risen and their tops are golden.

5. Serve with raspberries.

Each serving contains 2.8gnet carbs, 7.7g fat, and 8.8g protein.

Berry Parfait

Makes 4 servings

Ingredients

4 splenda packets

3 teaspoons vanilla extract

30g raspberries

300g Greek yogurt

12 tablespoons whipped cream

6 fresh strawberries

Directions

1. Puree half of the raspberries and strawberries with half of the Splenda in a blender.

2. Roughly chop the leftover raspberries and add it to the puree.

3. Mix cream, vanilla extract and remaining Splenda in a bowl using an electric beater until soft peaks start to form.

4. Add yogurt to it and beat to stiffen the peaks.

5. and Place alternate layers of cream filling, and berry mixture in parfait glasses. Top with the leftover strawberries. Serve.

This dessert makes a great breakfast option as well.

Each serving contains 8.1g net carbs, 21.3g fat, and 15.8g protein.

Tiramisu

Yields 6 servings

Ingredients

5 egg whites

125g protein powder

25g dark unsweetened cocoa powder

350g mascarpone cheese

25 drops liquid sweetener

6 shots espresso

Directions

1. Beat egg whites in a bowl.

2. Add 75g protein powder to the egg whites along with 20g cocoa powder.

3. Add 10 drops of the sweetener and 150g mascarpone cheese to it and mix well.

4. Pour the mixture onto a non-stick baking tray that is 25cm long. Bake in a preheated oven to about 170 degrees Centigrade for around 15 to 20 minutes. Let it cool.

5. Blend the remaining mascarpone cheese with 50g protein powder. Add 10 drops of the sweetener to it and mix well. This is the topping.

6. Divide the cake base amongst six glass bowls. Pour espresso sweetened using five drops of the sweetener over it and then add the topping to it. Garnish it with the leftover cocoa powder and serve.

Each serving contains 2.7g net carbs, 28g protein, and 29g fat.

Chocolate Ricotta Pudding

Yields 6 servings

Ingredients

2 tablespoons butter

4 teaspoon Stevia

½ teaspoon cream of tartar

2 teaspoons vanilla extract

100ml single cream

4 eggs

200g dark chocolate with 85% cocoa

200g ricotta cheese

Directions

1. Preheat the oven to about 180 degrees Centigrade.

2. Separate the egg whites from the yolks.

3. Put the chocolate, egg yolks, cream, vanilla extract and ricotta in a bowl. Mix well together.

4. Put the egg whites in another bowl along with the cream of tartar. Beat using an electric beater until soft peaks start to form. Add in Stevia.

5. Fold in the egg white mixture in the chocolate mixture and mix well.

6. Melt butter in a pan and when it turns brown, put the chocolate mixture in the pan. Cook it for about two minutes.

7. Put it in the oven and bake for about 25 minutes. Serve it warm with ice cream.

Each serving contains 10g net carbs, 13.1g protein, and 27.3g fat.

Keto Cupcakes

Yields 7 servings

Ingredients

120g vanilla flavoured protein powder

200ml unsweetened coconut milk

90g unsweetened coconut flakes

4 tablespoons coconut oil

2 tablespoons Psyllium husk

20g dark chocolate with 85% cocoa

Directions

1. Mix protein powder with psyllium and coconut flakes in a bowl.

2. Add coconut oil and coconut milk to it and mix well.

3. Divide this batter into seven cupcake forms and fill them with the batter.

4. Crush the chocolate and then melt it. Decorate the cupcakes with the chocolate.

5. Freeze the cupcakes for half an hour and then store them in the fridge for a couple of hours. Serve and enjoy.

Each cupcake contains 10.1g net carbs, 17.15g protein, and 30.7g fat.

Cherry Cobbler

Yields 8 servings

Ingredients

2 ¼ cups low carb baking mix

¼ teaspoon of pure almond extract

3 cups of pitted sweet cherries

1 large egg

2 tablespoons of cultured sour cream

1/3 cup of heavy cream

3 tablespoons of unsalted butter stick

¼ teaspoon of salt

¾ teaspoon of cinnamon

½ cup of sucralose based sweetener

¼ cup of halved pecans

Directions

1. Start by making the biscuit. Use a food processor to pulse ½ teaspoon of cinnamon, 2 tablespoons of sucralose based sweetener, pecans, baking mix and salt until medium ground.

2. Add in the butter and pulse until the mixture resembles a coarse meal.

3. In a bowl, whisk the egg, sour cream and heavy cream. Transfer the mixture into the food processor and pulse until everything is combined. You should end up with a dough. Pat it into a flat disk and then cover it with some plastic wrap and let it sit for 1-2 hours.

4. Preheat your oven to 400 degrees F.

5. Make the filling. Put ¼ teaspoon of cinnamon, almond extract, 1/3 cup of sucralose based sweetener and cherries in a medium bowl and mix. Transfer the mixture into a baking dish.

6. Divide the dough into 8 pieces and pat them until they are disk-like. Place the pieces of dough on top of the filling in the baking sheet and then bake for 35-40 minutes or until the fruits start bubbling and the biscuits start browning.

7. Serve with fresh whipped cream and enjoy.

Each serving contains 10.7g protein, 12.9g fat and 1.3g net carbs.

Toasted Rice and dates

Yields 48

Ingredients

1 cup of shredded coconut

2 cups of toasted rice cereals

1 teaspoon of vanilla extract

1/8 teaspoon of salt

1 ½ cups of chopped pitted dates

½ cup of sucralose based sweetener

¼ cup of unsalted butter

Directions

1. Mix the butter, dates and sweetener in a large saucepan and cook while constantly stirring for 8-15 minutes or until the dates are soft and the butter is melted. The mixture should form a brown sticky mass.

2. Add in coconut, cereal, vanilla and salt to the mixture and combine mix. Let the mixture cool down for a couple of minutes.

3. Once the mixture has cooled down, use your hands to squeeze and roll the mixture into 1 inch balls.

4. Set the balls on a wax paper-lined baking sheet and then chill until firm. Serve and enjoy. If you want to eat later, place the balls in an airtight container and refrigerate it for up to 1 week.

Each serving contains 10g net carbs, 2g fat and 0g protein.

Low-Carb Snack Recipes

Here are some wonderful low-carb snack recipes for you to munch on whenever hunger strikes.

Almond, Butter and Celery

Yields 1 serving

Ingredients

2 tablespoons almond butter

1 celery stalk

Directions

1. Cut the celery stalk into two to three pieces.
2. Smear the almond butter on the celery sticks and enjoy.

Each serving contains 6.2g net carbs, 13.7g protein, and 35.7g fat.

Cheese and Avocado

Yields 1 serving

Ingredients

30g cheddar cheese

½ avocado

Directions

1. Slice the avocado and serve it with cheese. Enjoy this quick and delicious snack.

Each serving contains 1.3g net carbs, 16.5g fat, and 6.4g protein.

Ginger Cookies

Yields 4 servings

Ingredients

¼ teaspoon of sea salt

1 ¼ teaspoons of ground ginger

1 ¼ teaspoons of ground cinnamon

2 teaspoons of baking soda

2 cups of sifted whole-wheat

4 tablespoons of molasses

1 large egg

1 ½ cups of natural sweetener

2/3 cup of canola oil

Directions

1. Preheat your oven to 350 degrees F.

2. Mix the sweetener and oil in a large bowl. Add in the egg and beat the mixture until combined. Add in molasses and stir until everything is well incorporated.

3. Mix the dry ingredients by sifting flour, ginger, cinnamon, baking soda and salt in a bowl. Give them a good mix and then transfer these into the wet ingredients. Stir until the mixture combines and forms dough.

4. Use your hands to roll the dough into 1-inch balls. Place the remaining ½ cup of sweetener in a small bowl and then roll the balls into it before you lay them down on an ungreased baking sheet. The balls should be an inch apart from each other.

5. Place the baking sheet in the oven and bake the cookies for 10-12 minutes or until soft. Transfer them to a wire rack once they are done and let them cool.

6. Serve and enjoy. These cookies can last up to 5 days when stored in an airtight container at room temperature.

Each cookie contains 15g carbs, 1g protein and 5g fat.

Baked Meatballs

Yields 8 meatballs

Ingredients

2 pounds of ground pork

1 large egg

1 tablespoon of grainy mustard

1 cup of fresh parsley leaves

1 tablespoon of ground black pepper

1 tablespoon of ground paprika

1 tablespoon of caraway seeds

½ tablespoon of salt

1 clove of minced garlic

Directions

1. Preheat your oven to 400 degrees F.

2. Take a large baking sheet and cover it with aluminum foil.

3. Mix the egg, mustard, parsley, pepper, paprika, caraway seeds, salt and garlic in a large bowl.

4. Add in the pork into the bowl and use your hands to knead it with the other ingredients. All ingredients should be well incorporated in the pork once you are done.

5. Moisten your hands by washing them in water and then shake off the excess water. Take a spoon, scoop a level tablespoon of pork, and then use your moist palms to roll the pork into a ball before placing the meatball into the prepared baking sheet. Repeat the whole process until all the ground pork is rolled into meatballs. The meatballs should be placed ½ inch apart on the baking sheet.

6. Place the baking sheet in the oven and let the meatballs bake for 20-25 minutes or until golden brown.

Remove from the oven and let them cool for a few minutes before you serve them.

Each meatball contains 6.6g fats, 2.9g of carbs and 41.5 g protein.

Crispy Tomato Chips

Yields 6 servings

Ingredients

2 tablespoons of grated Parmesan cheese

2 tablespoons of fresh chopped parsley

1 teaspoon of garlic powder

2 teaspoons of sea salt

2 tablespoons of extra virgin olive oil

6 cups thinly sliced beefsteak tomatoes.

Directions

1. Preheat your oven to about 200 degrees F.

2. Coat the sliced tomatoes with olive oil.

3. Lay the coated slices of tomatoes on a baking pan or onto a dehydrator shelve. Make sure that the tomatoes don't overlap each other.

4. In a small bowl, whisk together the grated parmesan cheese, parsley, garlic powder and sea salt. Make sure everything is well combined.

5. Scoop the mixture and sprinkle it over each slice of tomato.

6. If you are dehydrating, the process may take you 12-24 hours depending on the thickness of your tomato slices.

7. If you are baking, it will take you 4-5 hours for the tomato chips to be done. Constantly check the tomatoes after 30 minutes to see if the edges have started charring. Once they do, remove from the oven and let them cool for about 5 minutes. Serve and enjoy.

Each tomato chip contains 5.8g fats, 2.5g proteins and 2.1g carbs.

Conclusion

Thank you again for downloading this book!

I hope this book was able to help you learn about the low carb diet.

The next step is to implement what you have learnt.

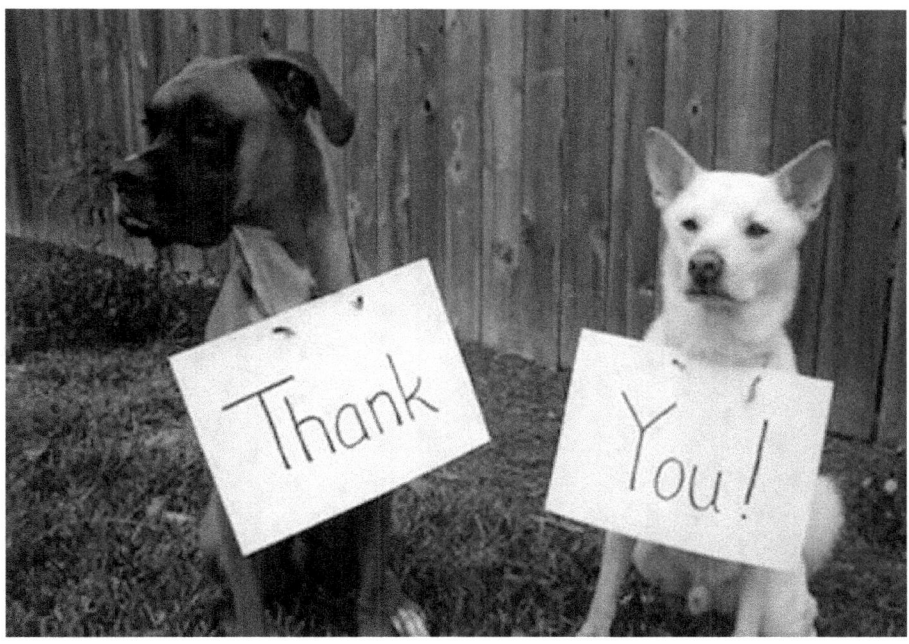

Finally, if you enjoyed this book, would you be kind enough to leave a review for this book on Amazon?

Thank you and good luck!

www.ingramcontent.com/pod-product-compliance
Lightning Source LLC
Chambersburg PA
CBHW062015280526
45787CB00005B/2109